Carla P. H. Alves Ribeiro César
Aline Cabral Oliveira
Silvia Baldrighi

Mouth breathing and its implications for development

Carla P. H. Alves Ribeiro César
Aline Cabral Oliveira
Silvia Baldrighi

Mouth breathing and its implications for development

The importance of prevention

ScienciaScripts

Imprint

Cover image: www.ingimage.com

This book is a translation from the original published under ISBN 978-3-639-74478-1.

Publisher:
Sciencia Scripts
is a trademark of
Dodo Books Indian Ocean Ltd. and OmniScriptum S.R.L publishing group

120 High Road, East Finchley, London, N2 9ED, United Kingdom
Str. Armeneasca 28/1, office 1, Chisinau MD-2012, Republic of Moldova, Europe
Managing Directors: Ieva Konstantinova, Victoria Ursu
info@omniscriptum.com

Printed at: see last page
ISBN: 978-620-8-60219-2

Carla Patrícia Hernandez Alves Ribeiro César (Organiser) / 2017

Editorial

This scientific book was written by many hands: hard-working, reflective and, above all, eager to contribute to a polysemic topic: mouth breathing.

A common complaint in speech therapy and otorhinolaryngology, its consequences extend to other areas and, for this reason, it is still a subject of research interest for many professionals.

This book therefore aims to highlight the impact of mouth breathing, especially in childhood, given that various aspects can be compromised and jeopardise the lives of children who breathe through their mouths.

I wish you all an excellent read and hope that the topics discussed here can clarify doubts, contribute to the work of professionals involved with this problem in their daily lives and perhaps instigate future research.

Yours sincerely,

Carla Patrícia Hernandez Alves Ribeiro César

Speech therapist

University lecturer - Federal University of Sergipe, Speech and Hearing Therapy Course, campus Prof. Antônio Garcia Filho, Lagarto, Sergipe, Brazil.

PhD in Human Communication Disorders from the Federal University of São Paulo, São Paulo, Brazil

Post-doctoral student in Emotional Facial Expressions at Fernando Pessoa University, Porto, Portugal.

Employees

Aline Cabral de Oliveira

PhD (Federal University of São Paulo, São Paulo, Brazil), MD (University of São Paulo,

Ribeirão Preto, São Paulo, Brazil), Speech and Hearing Therapist, Professor of Speech and Hearing Therapy, Federal University of Sergipe, campus Prof. Antônio Garcia Filho, Lagarto, Sergipe, Brazil.

Bárbara Cristina da Silva Rosa

PhD student and Master's degree (Pontifical Catholic University of São Paulo, São Paulo, Brazil), Speech and Hearing Therapist, Lecturer in the Speech and Hearing Therapy course at the Federal University of Sergipe, Prof. Antônio Garcia Filho campus, Lagarto, Sergipe, Brazil.

Carla Patrícia Hernandez Alves Ribeiro César

Post-doctoral student (Fernando Pessoa University, Porto, Portugal), MD (Federal University of São Paulo, São Paulo, Brazil), Speech and Hearing Therapist, Professor of Speech and Hearing Therapy at the Federal University of Sergipe, campus Prof. Antônio Garcia Filho, Lagarto, Sergipe, Brazil.

Caroline Oliveira dos Santos Menezes

Clinical speech therapist, graduated from the Federal University of Sergipe, campus Prof. Antônio Garcia Filho, Lagarto, Sergipe, Brazil.

Jucimara Nascimento Gois

Clinical speech therapist, graduated from the Federal University of Sergipe, campus Prof. Antônio Garcia Filho, Lagarto, Sergipe, Brazil.

Priscila Silva Passos

Master's Degree (Pontifical Catholic University of São Paulo, São Paulo, Brazil), Clinical Speech Therapist, graduated from the Federal University of Sergipe, São Cristóvão campus, São Cristóvão, Sergipe, Brazil.

Sílvia Elaine Zuim de Moraes Baldrighi

MD (Federal University of São Paulo, São Paulo, Brazil), Speech and Hearing Therapist, Professor of Speech and Hearing Therapy, Federal University of Sergipe, São Cristóvão campus, São Cristóvão, Sergipe, Brazil.

Sonia Coelho

PhD student (Fernando Pessoa University, Porto, Portugal), Master (Pontifical Catholic University of São Paulo, São Paulo, Brazil), Speech Therapist and CEO of +Expressão in Porto, Portugal.

Thaynara Alves dos Santos

Clinical phonoaudiologist, graduated from the Federal University of Sergipe, Prof. Dr. G. G. L., campus of the Federal University of Sergipe.
Antônio Garcia Filho, Lagarto, Sergipe, Brazil.

Summary

CHAPTER 1

Phonoaudiological assessment and treatment of altered respiratory mode

Carla Patrícia Hernandez Alves Ribeiro César

Jucimara Nascimento Gois

Caroline Oliveira dos Santos Menezes

Bárbara Cristina da Silva Rosa

Sílvia Elaine Zuim de Moraes Baldrighi

Mouth breathing is a concern for health specialists, especially speech therapists, because its alterations can have negative effects on an individual's development, especially in childhood. It should be emphasised, however, that sequelae alter quality of life (QoL) depending on their onset, duration of the problem and chronicity[1].

QoL is generally affected in respiratory disorders caused by asthma, due to dyspnoea[2] and can therefore generate respiratory discomfort; in physical activities associated with speech and oral emissions that require greater vocal intensity[3], as well as changes in chewing, swallowing and speech patterns - regardless of the severity of the asthma condition[4] and in sleep quality[2]. In addition, chronic and progressive respiratory diseases can cause behavioural, cardiovascular and neurological changes[5], directly affecting QoL, as in obstructive sleep apnoea syndrome - OSAS6, and there may also be overlapping neurocognitive disorders in patients with this condition[7]. Therefore, preventive measures need to be planned and implemented to improve the living conditions of these individuals[8].

The literature has pointed out its effects on speech, socialisation and academic performance, making its early detection and the planning and implementation of preventive measures essential to minimise its sequelae[9].

In this sense, actions in educational and health institutions are still lacking in this regard, since 12% of parents and 35% of educators said they knew about and identified mouth breathing[10].

The following are some thoughts on speech therapy and assessment.

Assessment and Speech Therapy

The assessment begins with an interview or anamnesis, which should include the complaint and the history of this complaint, data on the subject's life history and their development in general. As some manifestations are common in mouth breathing, it is important to ask about sleep quality (including the application of the Epworth scale to check for excessive daytime sleepiness), snoring, lip and tongue posture in everyday life and during sleep, the presence of sialorrhoea (especially at night)[11], eating[12] and appetite - including the development and performance of other oral functions such as chewing, swallowing and speech; whether or not there is a loss of smell and taste; academic/labour performance (the latter in the case of adults); whether or not attention is maintained; whether or not there are behavioural problems; which specialists are monitoring the case and medications being used - for future contacts, among other questions specific to each case.

Because the respiratory mode alters different systems, it is ideal for the speech and hearing assessment to be complete, especially in children, and for other specialities to also complement the diagnosis, so that interdisciplinary measures can be adopted, especially with the otorhinolaryngologist, orthodontist[13], physiotherapist, allergist and nutritionist, if necessary.

Whatever method is adopted (assessment or therapy), it is recommended that the subject undergoing the procedure understands the procedures adopted and the reason for the tests to be carried out. When the process is carried out with adults, an initial dialogue about the possible causes and the tests to be carried out is essential.

With children, the process can be facilitated with images or stories, such as "Mouth-breathing Augustus", which in a simple way explains to the child the signs, symptoms, consequences, evaluation and therapy to improve the nasal breathing mode[14].

As the main complaint is altered breathing, we suggest starting the assessment with breathing. Observation begins in the waiting room, when you can see whether the patient has their mouth fully or partially open.

In clinical assessment, in addition to visual inspection of the oral and nasal cavities, simple procedures are used to check nasal airflow during exhalation. To do this, a metal mirror (Glatzel, Gertner or Altmann) can be used so that comparisons can be made between exhalations from both nostrils, checking for symmetry and permeability. To this end, we have used the Altmann millimetre mirror (from Prófono®), which should be used in an unrefrigerated environment and better detects nasal obstructions. Melo et al[15] have suggested the use of the Peak Nasal Inspiratory Flow (PNIF), a silicone instrument that also helps to detect possible nasal obstructions, but differs from the previous instrument in that it measures from a maximum/forceful nasal inspiration (Figure 1). Both instruments are easy to acquire and inexpensive, and mirrors have been found to discriminate nasal obstructions better than the PNIF[15]. Other instruments can be used and are more effective, such as active anterior rhinomanometry, acoustic rhinometry[16] and impulse/force oscillometry[17], but they are expensive.

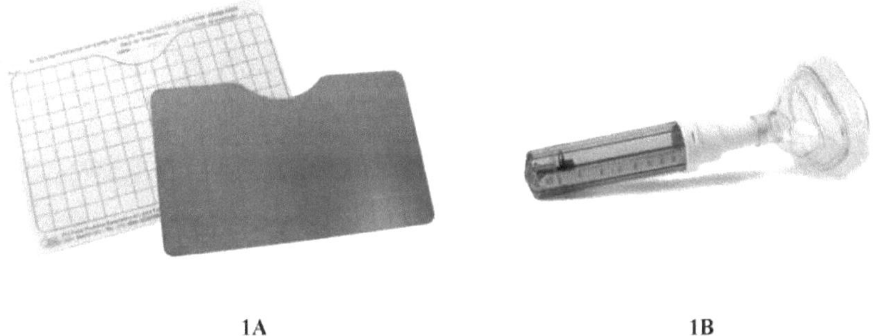

1A **1B**

Figura 1. Images of the usual instruments used to assess expiratory nasal airflow: 1A) Altmann's Millimetre Mirror and 1B) Peak Nasal Inspiratory Flow (PNIF).

It's worth pointing out, however, that research has shown that the Glatzel mirror doesn't seem to be a reliable tool for assessing nasal patency in the sample investigated, except in cases of severe nasal obstruction, i.e. surgical and allergic patients[18].

However, nasal airflow obtained in the mirror is still routinely used in speech therapy clinics and is classified considering the extent of its blurring in the mirror, being graded in six points:

1=no nasal airway leakage, 2=mild nasal airway leakage, 3=mild to moderate nasal airway leakage, 4=moderate nasal airway leakage, 5=moderate to intense nasal airway leakage and 6=intense nasal airway leakage[19] or by analysing the volume occupied by outlining the space in Autocad software[15]. If asymmetries or a reduction in expiratory nasal airflow are found, as well as a reduced time to maintain breathing through the nose (measured by a stopwatch), an otorhinolaryngological assessment is essential. In fact, speech therapy is only started once the etiological factor of the altered breathing mode has been eliminated (with the exception of rhinopathies).

As far as speech therapy assessment is concerned, language and speech can be assessed both informally, through spontaneous conversation or stimuli that instigate dialogue, and through objective tests, such as the use of word repetition or picture naming. Some protocols have been used, such as the MBGR20, AMIOFE21 and PAFORE22 - which have scores and can thus enable professionals to make comparisons over the course of sessions and qualitatively classify cervical orofacial myofunctional disorders into different degrees of severity - from high-grade to within normal standards[23].

In the case of children, the ideal is a comprehensive assessment, even if the complaint is just a change in breathing mode.

In order to directly investigate the signs and symptoms of mouth breathing (Index for Identifying the Signs and Symptoms of Mouth Breathing - IISSRO), the research group at the Federal University of Pernambuco, Recife, Brazil, developed this index, which contains information on breathing mode (thirteen items), signs related to breathing mode (observed in the assessment, with thirteen items), symptoms reported by carers or the patient themselves (six items), and if there are less than 50% of affirmative answers, the IISSRO indicates that there are no changes in breathing mode; 51 to 60 per cent is considered mixed; 61 to 79 per cent as mild mouth breathing; 80 to 89 per cent as moderate and 90 per cent upwards as severe mouth breathing[24].

And what are the main characteristics found in the speech of mouth breathers? Researchers[9] have shown tongue interposition in phonemes where the tongue should not behave this way (in Brazil, in words containing /t/, /d/, /n/ and /l/), distortion of the sounds /s/ and /J7 - known as lisping and articulatory changes.

Therefore, the repetition of a list of words and the naming of pictures are tests that are usually carried out, and it is important to record them on video in order to analyse the speech sample obtained in detail, as well as to advise the patient and their family of the changes found and future comparisons of the therapeutic measures adopted, verifying whether or not the therapeutic proposal has had the desired effect.

Awareness of the appropriate articulatory points and strengthening the muscles involved are objectives to be worked on in speech therapy sessions. Initially, in a direct way (with videos, proprioceptive clues, diagrams and drawings) until speech is worked on informally (games, storytelling and dialogues, for example), so that the articulatory patterns are automated by the patient.

As the posture of the lips and tongue change as a result of mouth breathing, being ajar/open and lowered, respectively[25, 26], these aspects should be observed during the assessment and subsequently incorporated into the therapeutic planning, including raising awareness of the correct posture of these structures and increasing tone by offering isometric exercises[27]. It should be emphasised that awareness is the key to any therapeutic process and is not readily acquired. It is necessary for the family to cooperate in this process and for the therapist to offer strategies to help the patient remember to keep the lips sealed and the apex of the tongue on the palatine papillae, depending on the patient's type of face. We recommend the use of stickers in different places, alarms that can be set off by mobile phone and even sending messages via whatsapp by the therapist with inspiring words such as: "you can keep your lips sealed" or even "if your tongue isn't on the papilla now, no problem, just do it now!" to facilitate this process.

Other social technologies have been mentioned in the literature that can help speech therapy, such as the use of the internet, which makes videos available, or the making of videos to explain the consequences of mouth breathing or the therapeutic path[28], as well as the use of different strategies for training nasal breathing and keeping the lips sealed, such as keeping spatulas and pieces of gelatine sheet between the lips, playful blowing activities, such as the use of mother-in-law's tongue and soap bubbles, for example.Another procedure that facilitates proprioception of the sealed lip posture is the use of an elastic bandage in the orbicular region of the mouth[27], as can be seen in figure 2. It should be changed every 48 hours or, in our experience, daily in very hot places.

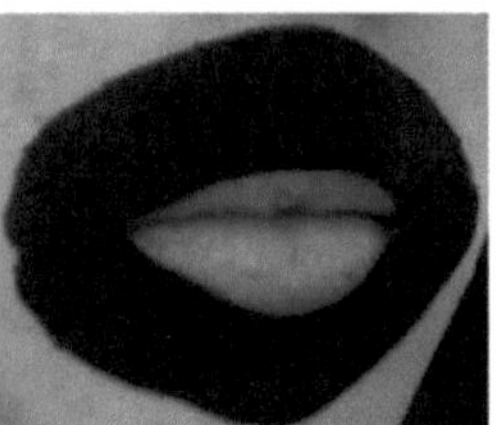

Figura 2. Elastic bandage fixed over the orbicularis of the mouth, with a neutral point in the middle of each bandage strip [personal collection].

Head posture is generally anteriorised in breathers, and this is also an aspect to be made aware of in the therapeutic process.

As the tongue muscles tend to decrease in tone in mouth breathers, another function that is compromised is swallowing[26], which generally shows the presence of compensatory movements, such as lip pressing.

Ideally, photographic documentation should be carried out in a standardised way, recording posture, face, occlusion and the intraoral cavity[30] and comparing the records throughout the therapeutic process, showing the patient and family (in the case of mouth-breathing children) the progress achieved.

Speech therapy has beneficial effects and one of the concerns of family members, when the patients are children, is how long the patient will need to undergo speech therapy. Thus, some authors have reported varying times, since the procedures/methods used differ, but we have compiled the results obtained from the literature, as can be seen in the table below (Table 1).

Table 1. Therapeutic procedures adopted and time taken to discharge patients due to the introduction of nasal breathing.

Researchers	Speech therapy proposal	Time to restore nasal breathing
Gallo; Campioto[jl]	Guidance (for carrying out the exercises at home) and application of orofacial myofunctional exercises, nasal breathing	10 sessions

	training, among others.	
Lourenço; César[12]	Training and awareness of nasal breathing; inspection of expiratory nasal airflow before and after the application of exercises; manoeuvres manoeuvres warming up and vascularisation of the orofacial muscles; nasal hygiene; orofacial myofunctional exercises and guidance.	Between 3 and 6 sessions (average: 5 sessions)
Marson et al."	Training and awareness of nasal breathing; manoeuvres to warm up and vascularise the orofacial musculature; application of points and motor zones on the face; passive manoeuvres; use of the distal impulse; myofunctional exercises and recording patients' perceptions of their olfactory conditions and nasal obstructions.	12 sessions
Average		**Nine sessions**

Other aspects that may be altered in mouth breathers concern the structural aspects of the hard palate, making it either narrow or deep or both, most likely as a result of the tongue being lowered to the floor of the mouth; and dental occlusion, leading to orthodontic changes[25] and a tendency towards a more elongated facial growth pattern[34]. These aspects are detailed in greater depth in another chapter of this book and deserve special attention from orthodontists when it comes to assessment and treatment.

In addition to what has been said about the process of assessment and speech therapy for mouth-breathing patients, the Motrisis® application (CTS Informática) has been successfully used in Brazil for different alterations in orofacial motricity. This software can be used to record anamnesis, assessment and therapy, as there are playful strategies for the patient to achieve the therapeutic objectives proposed by the speech therapist, such as performing isometric, isotonic and nasal breathing awareness exercises.

Conclusion

Intervention to reorganise nasal breathing is multimodal and complex, as it depends on the work of different health specialists, and it is important to share knowledge and work in an interdisciplinary way.

References

1. César CPHAR, Silva KD, Paranhos LR, Baldrighi SEZDM. Quality of life of subjects with and without nose breathing difficulties. Biosci. J. 2016; 32(1): 272-8.

2. Tomaz RR. Does the mouth breathing pattern affect sleep quality, respiratory function and functional capacity in asthmatic children? 2014. 67f. Master's Degree [Postgraduate Programme in Physiotherapy], Universidade Federal do Rio Grande do Norte, Natal, Rio Grande do Norte, Brazil.

3. Campanha SMA, Fontes MJF, Santos JLFD. Dyspnoea in individuals with asthma, allergic rhinitis and mouth breathing. Rev. CEFAC 2012; 14(2): 268-73.

4. Castro MSJ, Toro AADC, Sakano E, Ribeiro JD. Evaluation of orofacial functions of the stomatognathic system and respiratory mode in asthma severity levels. J Soc Bras Fonoaudiol. 2012;24(2): 119-24.

5. Silva ADLD, Catão MHCV, Costa RO, Costa IRRS. Multidisciplinarity in sleep apnoea: a literature review. Rev. CEFAC. 2014; 16(5):1621-6.

6. Lacerda VMA, Cunha ACR, Souza IR, Santos Vasconcelos R, Melo LTM, Abdon APV. Quality of life (QOL) and clinical aspects of patients with obstructive sleep apnoea syndrome (OSAS) being treated with continuous positive airway pressure (CPAP). Brazilian Journal of Quality of Life 2013; 5(1): 22-30.

7. Hilario SM, Silva EVCM, Chiloff CLM, Magalhães Bertoz AP, Micheletti KR, Cuoghi OA, Weber SAT. Neuropsychological disorders and Sleep Apnoea Syndrome in children. Arch Health Invest 2014, 3(3): 65-75.

8. Santos JC, Granzotti RBG, Oliveira Barreto AC, Oliveira CC, Silva K, Moraes Baldrighi SEZ, César CPHAR. Little Citizen Project: health promotion and prevention of eating disorders and orofacial myofunctional disorders in preschoolers. Common Disorders. 2016; 28(1): 151-61.

9. Hitos SF, Arakaki R, Solé D, Weckx LL. Oral breathing and speech disorders in children.

J Paediatr 2013; 89(4): 361-5.

10. Borges ERS. Parents' and educators' perceptions of mouth breathing. 82f. 2014. Master's Degree [Dental Sciences], University of Alfenas, Minas Gerais, Brazil.

11. Costa MD, Valentim AF, Becker HMG, Motta AR. Multiprofessional assessment findings of mouth-breathing children. Rev. CEFAC 2015; 17(3): 864-78.

12. Brandão Canuto MS, Batista de Moura J, Lira dos Anjos CA. Food preferences of mouth breathers in a primary school. Rev. CEFAC 2016; 18(4): 811-7.

13. Baldrighi SEZM, César CPHAR, Brito AFD, Ferreira GG, Rodrigues MRC, Nascimento LT, Santos FS. Orofacial myofunctional profile of children treated at the

paediatric dental outpatient clinic at the Aracaju/SE University Hospital. Distúrbios Comun. 2015; 27(1): 85-96.

14. Santos CS, César CPHAR. Augusto mouth breather. São Paulo: Gearte; 2016.

15. Melo DL, Santos RVM, Castro Perilo TV, Becker HMG, Motta AR. Assessment of mouth breathers: use of the Glatzel mirror and peak nasal inspiratory flow. CoDAS 2013;25(3):236-41.

16. Pérez AO. Validation of nasal inspiratory flow determination. Allergol Inmunol Clin. 2004;19:25-8.

17. Andrade FMD. Study of respiratory system compliance in obese individuals with different levels of body mass index using impulse oscillometry. 87f. 2008. Master's Degree [Biological Sciences], Federal University of Pernambuco, Recife, Brazil.

18. Bassi IB, Franco LP, Motta AR. Efficacy of using the Glatzel mirror to assess nasal patency. Rev Soc Bras Fonoaudiol. 2009;14(3):367-71.

19. Trindade IEK, Trindade Junior AS, Teixeira ACMS, Fukushiro AP, Silva ASCD, Araújo BMAM, Trindade-Suedam IK, Genaro KF, Yamashita RP. Instrumental assessment of velopharyngeal function, breathing and mastication. Course on Congenital Lip and Palate Anomalies, 46; 2013.

20. Marchesan IQ, Berretin-Felix G, Genaro KF. MBGR Protocol of orofacial myofunctional evaluation with scores. Int J Orofacial Myology. 2012; 38:77-38.

21. Felício CM, Ferreira CL. Protocol of orofacial myofunctional evaluation with scores. Int J of Pediatr Otorhinolaryngol. 2008; 72(3):367-75.

22. Susanibar F, Dacillo C. Protocol for the phonoaudiological assessment of breathing with scores - PAFORE. São José dos Campos: Pulso Editorial; 2013.

23. Santos C, Amaral AKFJ, Soares JFR. Software for Myofunctional Classification in the Speech and Hearing Clinic. J. Health Inform. 2016; 8(5): 157-63.

24. Melo ACC. Nasal geometry pre- and post-cleaning technique in mouth-breathing children. 114f. 2015. Master's Degree [Human Communication Health], Federal University of Pernambuco, Recife, Brazil.

25. Pacheco AB, Silva AMT, Mezzomo CL, Berwig LC, Neu AP. The relationship between mouth breathing and non-nutritive sucking habits and alterations in the stomatognathic system. Rev. Cefac 2012; 14(2): 281-9.

26. Andrade-Balieiro FB, Azevedo R, Chiari BM. Aspects of the stomatognathic system pre- and post-adenotonsillectomy. CoDAS 2013; 25(3): 229-35.

27. César CPHAR, Trench JA, Nascimento GKBO, Sordi C. Mouth breathing: speech therapy intervention and the limits of treatment - part II. In: Nahsan FPS, Sordi C, Paranhos LR (Org.). Coletâneas em saúde. São José dos Pinhais: Editora Plena; 2015b. p. 67-77.

28. César CPHAR, Domenis DR, Silva K, Guedes-Granzotti RB, Dornelas R, Pellicani AD. The use of social technologies in Speech and Hearing Therapy - an experience report from the Speech and Hearing Therapy Course at the Federal University of Sergipe, Lagarto - SE. In: Nahsan FPS, Sordi C, Paranhos LR, organisers. Health collections. São José dos Pinhais: Editora Plena; 2015a. 3v. p. 79-90.

29. Bezerra LA. Cervical symmetry and its relationship with masticatory preference side in children with mouth breathing secondary to allergic rhinitis. 197f. 2014. Master's Degree (Health Sciences), Federal University of Pernambuco, Recife, Brazil.

30. César CPHAR, Sordi C, Baldrighi SEZM, Trench JA, Nascimento GKBO. Mouth breathing: speech therapy intervention and the limits of treatment - part I. In: Sordi C, Nahsan FPS, Paranhos LR, organisers. Health collections. São José dos Pinhais: Editora Plena; 2015c. 2v. p. 65-78.

31. Gallo J, Campiotto AR. Orofacial myofunctional therapy in mouth breathing children. Rev. CEFAC 2009;11(Suppl 3):305-10.

32. Lourenço CT, César CPHAR. Phonoaudiological rehabilitation of the oral breathing mode: therapeutic time In: XIII Congresso Metodista de Iniciação e Produção Científica, 2010, São Bernardo do Campo. Methodist Scientific Congress. São Bernardo do Campo: Methodist University of São Paulo; 2010.

33. Marson A, Tessitore A, Sakano E, Nemr K. Effectiveness of speech therapy and proposal for brief intervention in mouth breathers. Rev CEFAC 2012; 14: 1153-66.

34. Berwig LC, Marquezan M, Trevisan ME, Chiodelli L, Rubim ADBP, Corrêa ECR, Silva AMTD. Facial anthropometric measurements according to diagnosis of breathing mode and gender in adults. Rev. CEFAC 2015; 17(6): 1882-8.

CHAPTER 2

Auditory Processing in Mouth Breathers

Aline Cabral de Oliveira

Priscila Silva Passos

Thaynara Alves dos Santos

The auditory system (AS) is made up of the sensory organ of hearing, the auditory pathways of the nervous system and brain structures that receive, analyse and interpret sound information[1] and is often required in communication situations. This system can be divided into two distinct but interrelated parts, defined as the central and peripheral auditory systems. The peripheral portion comprises the structures of the outer, middle and inner ears and the peripheral nervous system (the vestibulo-cochlear nerve)[2] and the central portion refers to the auditory pathways located in the brainstem and cortical areas[3].

This system is fully formed at birth, and the auditory pathways need to be matured through sound stimulation. The critical period of hearing, i.e. from birth to two years of age, corresponds to the period of greatest neuronal plasticity of the auditory pathways. At this time, the auditory system can be modified depending on the quantity and quality of external stimuli received. The richer the auditory stimuli, the greater the number of connections between the inner ear and the cortex[4]. Children who do not receive adequate auditory stimulation during the first two or three years of life will probably not have their language potential fully developed.

The first few years of a baby's life are full of learning and it is through auditory feedback that the basic concepts necessary for the construction of language are formed, organised into various neuropsychological, organic and affective processes, enabling symbolic learning[5]. Hearing, as a special sense, comes later, as the child stores all kinds of information indistinctly. Sounds begin to have real meaning when the process of learning to hear is established, a process that can be influenced by the environment[6]. The integrity of the auditory system is essential for the acquisition and development of oral language, as this is a prerequisite, since children must be able to pay attention, detect, discriminate, localise sounds, memorise and integrate auditory experiences in order to be able to recognise and understand speech[7].

However, some people do not have complete integrity of the auditory system and the impact of this sensory deprivation is significant, because it not only affects the ability to properly understand sound information, but mainly the way they relate to their environment and culture. There are countless alterations related to the sensory organ of hearing that can cause biological, social and even psychological impacts[8-9], among which we highlight middle ear infections.

These infections, called Otitis Media (OM), for example, are very common diseases in childhood. They are characterised by inflammation, which can be accompanied by effusion, i.e. a collection of fluid in the middle ear space. It is an infection that primarily affects infants and young children, and is less frequent in older children, adolescents and adults. It is one of the most prevalent infectious diseases worldwide: more than 80 per cent of children suffer an episode of acute otitis media (AOM) before the age of three and 40 per cent will have had six or more recurrences by the age of seven[10]. Otitis media with effusion is one of the most common diseases in children, affecting between 28 and 38 per cent of the pre-school population[11].

Dysfunction or malfunction of the auditory tube (AT) plays an important role in the aetiology of otitis media[12]. Otitis media with effusion is the most common cause of conductive hearing loss in children and has become increasingly common in recent years. According to some authors, there are several causes of otitis media, but the malfunctioning of the auditory tube, causing the middle ear not to ventilate, seems to be the most widely accepted[13-14].

The Eustachian tube is a structure that connects the tympanic cavity of the middle ear to the nasopharynx and has the basic function of ventilation, allowing the pressure in the middle ear to be equalised with the pressure in the environment. It also provides drainage of middle ear secretions into the nasopharynx and protects it from contaminated secretions[11-13-14]. This tube measures between 31 and 38 mm in length and is inclined at 45 degrees in adults, but is more horizontal in children[15-16].

This practically horizontal characteristic of AT can favour the entry of liquids into the middle ear and, consequently, the onset of OM, depending on the posture in which the child is breastfed or receives food from a bottle.

The junction of the bony and cartilaginous portions forms the isthmus of the auditory tube which, similar to a valve, controls the entry of air[17]. The ET is closed at rest and through the action of the soft palate tensor and soft palate levator muscles, which are activated when swallowing and/or yawning, air passes from the nasal part of the pharynx to the middle ear. This allows the pressure of the external air to be equalised with the pressure in the tympanic cavity and also aerates the middle ear. This mechanism protects the ear from rapid pressure changes, keeps the mucosa preserved and allows the tympano-ossicular unit to vibrate without complications[18-19].

Children who have an oral respiratory mode due to alterations in the nasal septum, adenoid hyperplasia, inflamed tonsils, hypertrophic nasal conchae and/or allergic rhinitis[20] may have alterations in the pressure level in the middle ear, which can be a determining factor in the development of otitis media and, consequently, alterations in hearing[21]. Tonsil hypertrophy and swelling of the nasal mucosa can cause the auditory tube to malfunction, making it difficult to regulate pressure, which can be a predictor of otitis media[22-23].

In this way, mouth-breathing children become vulnerable to frequent variations in hearing thresholds, making it difficult to form acoustic patterns, which can result in (Central) Auditory Processing Disorders, a hearing disorder characterised by the inability to analyse and interpret sound patterns.

The degradation of the auditory signal can cause impairments in speech understanding in noisy environments, changes in auditory memory, binaural integration and temporal processes[24]. In one study, the authors observed in Dutch schoolchildren that otitis media associated with fluctuating hearing loss in childhood affects speech perception skills[25].

Failure to establish acoustic patterns can jeopardise attention, concentration and the development of important auditory skills[26]. These skills are associated with adequate speech perception, the process of developing communication and learning to read and write. These skills depend on the maturation and integrity of the auditory pathways, which can be compromised in patients with altered respiratory mode[27-28].

(Central) auditory processing refers to the mechanisms and processes that occur in the auditory system, responsible for behavioural phenomena such as [29]:

L Sound localisation and lateralisation - the former is the ability to identify where the sound originates and lateralisation, in turn, is related to the behaviour of localising sounds to the right and left, with the individual's head as a reference[30-31]. Alterations in these abilities prevent the individual from identifying the direction of the sound source;
D Auditory discrimination - is the act of differentiating between two or more sound stimuli[32]. Alterations in this type of ability cause learning difficulties and often occur in schoolchildren who have difficulty discriminating between two phonemes with similar sounds;
R Recognition of auditory patterns - is the ability to identify the sound and the sound source with the ability to classify or name what they have heard[32].

A Temporal aspects of hearing (temporal resolution, temporal masking, temporal integration and temporal ordering) are skills that are closely related to the individual's ability to recognise, discern and perceive the segmental and suprasegmental aspects of speech[33-34]. Some of the alterations found in these skills are auditory related to prosody, rhythm, intonation and sound duration - which can later be associated with reading and writing. Children may have difficulties with punctuation rules as well as with reading itself.
D Auditory performance with competing acoustic signals - an ability that allows the subject to maintain attention to a sound, even in the presence of other sounds in the environment, with the sound that is paid attention to being called the figure and the other sounds being called the "background". When the auditory figure-to-ground ability is compromised, it makes it difficult for the student to pay attention, for example, to what the teacher is saying when there are parallel conversations in the room (competitive sound).
Difficulties in processing auditory information need to be detected early, as a failure in this ability can lead to information being interpreted in a distorted way. Individuals who complain of school difficulties generally perform worse in auditory processing tests due to delayed maturation of auditory skills[35]. Therefore, professionals who work with mouth breathers should also be aware of their patients' auditory development.

The impact of mouth breathing on auditory processing: research in the field

According to some authors, alterations in auditory processing are usually associated with common characteristics in these individuals, such as frequent tiredness and sleepiness, which can interfere with school performance and common childhood activities, such as playing games that require greater physical effort and attention, leading to delays in the development of these individuals[36].

In a study carried out to verify the occurrence of alterations in the auditory processing of mouth-breathing children, more alterations were found in the sequential memory tests for non-verbal sounds. The results indicate that altered breathing patterns are an important etiological factor in the emergence of auditory processing problems and, because of this, constant prevention should be sought for proper diagnosis and treatment[37].

Another study was carried out to identify the occurrence of alterations in verbal and non-verbal sequential memory, localisation and figure-ground tests in mouth-breathing children. Ten subjects of both genders took part in the study, divided into two groups: five mouth breathers and five nasal breathers. The Paediatric Speech Intelligibility test (PSI) and the Simplified Auditory Processing Assessment (ASPA) were applied. The results showed differences in the auditory localisation tests and the non-verbal sequential memory test between the groups[38].

Toniolo et al. observed that children between the ages of seven and ten with a history of otitis media in the first year of life and recurrent episodes in the pre-school and/or school years may have altered auditory processing. These children, when compared to others with no history of the condition, showed poorer performance in the auditory processes of monotic listening with low redundancy and verbal dichotic, as well as temporal resolution[39]. Monotic listening is related to tasks that use only one ear, while dichotic listening involves both ears to understand an auditory message[40].

Hitos et al. [41] found that in addition to factors such as sagging orofacial muscles, incorrect positioning of the tongue and other structures in the oral cavity (as mentioned in the previous chapter), breathing can be altered due to daytime sleepiness, poor cerebral oxygenation and immature auditory processing skills.

Conclusion

Considering the fact that the establishment of mouth breathing can negatively interfere with the auditory system and auditory maturation, thus affecting the development of auditory skills and learning, the importance of auditory assessment and auditory processing in the process of multidisciplinary care for mouth breathing children is emphasised.

In this way, professional action allows for the development of a more complete therapeutic approach that minimises alterations in the development of auditory function and, consequently, prevents speech and learning disorders in these individuals.

References

1- Momensohn-Santos TM, Dias AMN, Valente CHB, Assayag FM. Anatomy and physiology of the organ of hearing and balance. In: Momensohn-Santos TM, Russo ICP (Org.). Prática de audiologia clínica. 6. ed. São Paulo: Cortez; 2007. p. 12-44.

2- Bonaldi LV. Anatomical bases of hearing and balance. In: Boéchat EM (Org.). Tratado de audiologia. 2ed. Rio de Janeiro: Guanabara Koogan; 2015.

3- Haines D. Fundamental neuroscience. In: Boéchat EM (Org.). Tratado de audiologia. 2. ed. Rio de Janeiro: Guanabara Koogan; 2015.

4- Ramos BD. The importance of hearing in language development. In: Caldas N, Caldas SN, Sih T (Org.). Otology and audiology in paediatrics. Rio de Janeiro: Revinter; 1999. p. 168-71.

5- Marchiori LLM. Analysing Hearing Alterations in Schoolchildren with Complaints of Learning Problems. Fono Atual 2002; 21: 10-5.

6- Russo ICP, Santos TMM. Audiology for Children. São Paulo: Cortez; 1994.

7- Azevedo MF, Vieram RM, Vilanova, LCP. Hearing Development in Normal and High-Risk Children. São Paulo: Plexus; 1995.

8- Boéchat EM. Plasticity of the auditory system in terms of hearing sensitivity to pure tones and responses to speech in sensorineural hearing loss [thesis]. São Paulo: University of São Paulo Medical School; 2003.

9- Veiga LR, Merlo ARC, Mengue SS. Satisfaction with hearing aids in daily life in users of the Army health system. Braz J Otorhinolaryngol. 2005; 71(1): 67-73.

10- World Health Organisation. Primary ear and hearing care training resource; 2006 http://www.who.int/pbd/deafness/activities/hearingcare/advanced.pdf

11- Bluestone CD. Studies in otitis media: Children's Hospital of Pittsburgh- University of Pittsburgh progress report - 2004. Laryngoscope. 2004; 114(suppl 105): 1-26.

12- Corbeel L. What is new in otitis media? Eur J Pediatric. 2007; 166(6): 511-9.

13- Straetemans M, van Heerbeek N, Tonnaer E, Ingels KJ, Rijkers GT, Zielhuis GA. A comprehensive model for the aetiology of otitis media with effusion. Med Hypotheses. 2001; 57(16): 784-91.

14- Nguyen LH, Manoukian JJ, Tewfik TL, Sobol SE, Joubert P, Mazer BD et al. Evidence of allergic inflammation in the middle ear and nasopharynx in atopic children with otitis media with effusion. J Otolaryngol. 2004; 33(6): 345-51.

15- Sadler-Kimes D, Siegel MI, Todhunter JS. Age-related morphologic differences in the components of the eustachian tube/middle ear system. Ann Otol Rhinol Laryngol. 1989; 98(11): 854-8.

16- Ishijima K, Sando I, Balaban C, Suzuki C, Takasaki K. Length of the eustachian tube and its postnatal development: computer-aided three-dimensional reconstruction and measurement study. Ann Otol Rhinol Laryngol. 2000; 109(6): 542-8.

17- Rood SR, Doyle WJ. Anatomy: introduction. Ann Otol Rhinol Laryngol. 1985; 120 suppl 94: 6-8.

18- Bento RF, Miniti A, Marone SAM. Eustachian tube. In: Otology Treatise. São Paulo: EDUSP; 1998. p. 173-82.

19- Doyle WJ. Physiology: introduction. Ann Otol Rhinol Laryngol. 1995; 120 Suppl 94: 20-1.

20- Cintra CFSC, Castro FFM, Cintra PPVC. Orofacial alterations in mouth-breathing patients. Rev bras alergia imunopatol. 2000; 23(2): 78-83.

21- Braga MEL. Audiometric profile of chronic otitis media: analysis of 745 ears [dissertation]. Porto Alegre: Federal University of Rio Grande do Sul; 2014.

22- Ferraz MCA. Practical manual of oral motricity, assessment and treatment. Rio de

Janeiro: Revinter; 2001.

23- Lourenço EA, Lopes KC, Pontes Júnior A, Oliveira MH, Umemura A, Vargas AL. Comparative radiological and nasofibroscopic study of adenoid volume in mouth-breathing children. Rev Bras Otorrinolaringol. 2005; 71(1): 23-8.

24- Santos MFC, Ziliotto KN, Monteiro VG, Hirata CHW, Pereira LD, Weckx LLM. Evaluation of Central Auditory Processing in Children With and Without a History of Otitis Media. Brazilian Journal of Otorhinolaryngology. 2001; 67(4): 448-54.

25- Zumach A, Chenault MN, Anteunis LJC, Gerrits E. Speech Perception after Early-Life Otitis Media with Fluctuating Hearing Loss. Audiol Neurotol 2011; 16(5): 304-14.

26- Bianchini AP, Guedes ZCF, Hitos S. Mouth breathing: cause x hearing. Rev CEFAC. 2009; 11(1): 38-43.

27- Toffoli MB, Lamprecht RR. The stimulation of auditory-verbal skills in pre-syllabic children: contributions to the development of phonological awareness. Letras de Hoje. 2008; 43(3): 89-97.

28- Mendonça JE, Lemos SMA. Health promotion and phonoaudiological actions in early childhood education. Rev CEFAC. 2011; 13(6): 1017-30.

29- American Speech Language Hearing Association. Central auditory processing - current strategies and implications of clinical practice. Am J Audiology 1996; 5(2): 41-54.

30- Boothroyd A. Speech acoustics and perception. Austin (Texas): Pro-Ed; 1986.

31- Pereira LD and Cavadas M. Central auditory processing. In: Frota S. Fundamentos em fonoaudiologia - audiologia. Rio de Janeiro: Guanabara Koogan; 1998. p. 135-46.

32- Scaranello CA. Hearing rehabilitation after cochlear implantation. Medicina. 2005; 38(3/4): 273-8.

33- Muniz LF, Roazzi A, Schochat E, Teixeira CF, Lucena, JA. Evaluation of temporal resolution skills, using pure tone, in children with and without phonological disorders. Rev CEFAC. 2007; 9(4): 550-62.

34- Ishii C, Arashiro PM, Pereira LD. Temporal ordering and resolution in in-tune and out-of-tune professional and amateur singers. Pró-Fono Revista de Atualização Científica. 2006; 18 (3): 285-92.

35- Neves IF, Schochat E. Auditory processing maturation in children with and without school difficulties. Pró-Fono Rev Atual Cient. 2005; 17(3): 311-20.

36- Correa BM, Rossi AG, Roggia B, Silva AMT. Analysing the auditory skills of children with mouth breathing. Rev. CEFAC. 2011; 13(4): 668-75.

37- Netto ACD. Mouth breathing and central auditory processing disorders. In: Marchesan I, Zorzi J. Anuário CEFAC de fonoaudiologia - 1999/2000. Rio de Janeiro: Revinter. p. 259-78.

38- Macedo AM. Investigation of the central auditory skills of localisation, verbal and non-verbal sequential memory and figure-ground in mouth breathing children. [Monograph] Franca: University of Franca; 2003.

39- Villa PC. Verbal and temporal auditory skills in children aged 6 to 10 years with and without proven episodes of recurrent fluctuating conductive hearing loss in the first years of life (dissertation). Ribeirão Preto: University of São Paulo; 2014.

40- Toniolo IMF, Rossi AG, Borges ACLC, Pereira LD. Auditory processing: auditory ability of verbal and non-verbal sequential memory in schoolchildren. Rev Saúde. 1994; 20(3-4): 11-22.

41- Hitos SF, Arakaki R, Solé D, Weckx LL. Oral breathing and speech disorders in children. J Paediatr. 2013; 89: 361-5.

CHAPTER 3

Mouth breathing and learning: interrelationships

Caroline Oliveira dos Santos Menezes

Jucimara Nascimento Gois

Carla Patrícia Hernandez Alves Ribeiro César

Learning is a fundamental property of living beings, especially human beings, since we need to adapt to the environment in order to survive and interact. In this way, intrinsic and extrinsic factors have a significant impact on how we learn[1]. It therefore requires the intersection of several factors (Figure 1), according to the literature[2].

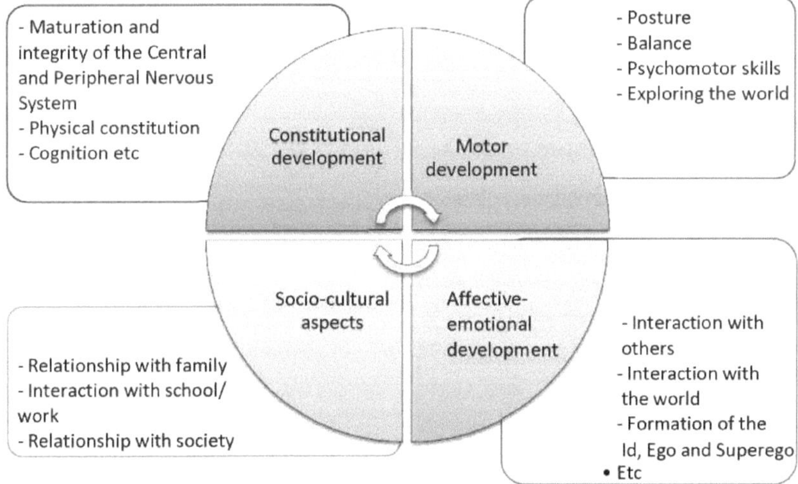

Figure 1. Factors that impact learning.

The aim of this chapter is not to go into all these aspects in depth, but to highlight mouth breathing as one of the constitutional factors that can impair learning, depending on how long it is present and how chronic it is.

A number of hypotheses have been put forward to explain the possibility of this negative correlation between difficulty in learning and altered respiratory mode, including sleep apnoea syndrome (OSAS) and obstructive airway factors and their possible impact on learning, as described below.

Obstructive sleep apnoea syndrome (OSAS)

OSAS is the most important and frequent respiratory sleep disorder[3]. It is characterised by the presence of daytime symptoms produced by five or more obstructive events of the apnoea and hypopnoea type per hour of sleep. Symptoms such as daytime hypersomnia, tiredness, feeling unwell, lack of attention, reduced memory, depression, decreased reflexes and a feeling of loss of organisational capacity are common complaints that should serve as a warning of the possible diagnosis of obstructive apnoea, when associated with complaints relating to nocturnal sleep[4].

Risk factors in childhood include obesity, tonsil hypertrophy (palatine or pharyngeal), craniofacial anomalies such as retrognathia and micrognathia[5], neuromuscular diseases[6], family history of tonsil hypertrophy[7], vitamin D depletion[8] and even genetic alterations involving TNF-a gene polymorphism, particularly -308G, which relates to the TNF-a cytokine, a glycopeptide related to intercellular reactions of tumour necrosis factor and, according to the literature[9], can regulate sleep.

There are several morbidity factors, including infections; endocrine, metabolic, nutritional, gastrointestinal, respiratory system, eye, ear, nose and throat diseases, among others, and in approximately 0.7 per cent of cases death can occur[10]. In addition to the above, the chances of a child with OSAS developing asthma may be around three times higher than in other children[11], as well as

sickle cell anaemia. This is because sickle cell anaemia can be considered a base disease for others, and knowledge of its biological aspects, cardiovascular implications and effects on the population's morbidity and mortality are important for understanding its real dimensions and, consequently, responding to the necessary demands related to public health, especially in relation to children, women and the elderly[12].

Despite the high incidence of OSAS in children, its diagnosis and treatment are challenges for public health due to the difficulty in objectively assessing its severity, and it is important to apply questionnaires to carers in order to investigate the clinical manifestations of OSAS, such as the Obstructive Sleep Apnea (OSA-18), which is made up of 18 questions divided into the following domains: sleep disorders, physical symptoms, emotional symptoms, daytime function and carer concerns, in order to investigate the impact of OSAS on children and their carers[13].

Therefore, health professionals need to know about OSAS and the care they should take when the patient is under their responsibility, especially in surgical circumstances. A study revealed that of the cases of death or permanent neurological sequelae following palatine tonsillectomy, 77% were children with OSAS, revealing that a validated paediatric risk assessment scoring system specific to OSAS needs to be developed in order to identify such children and thus adopt appropriate conduct[14].

Fleig[15] found an excessive delay in the diagnosis and treatment of OSAS in adult subjects who were followed up in a public referral hospital located in the south of Brazil, a fact that can compromise the quality of life of subjects affected by the disease. The same is true of its diagnosis in children, even in countries considered to be developed[16].

As such, the interdisciplinary team (such as paediatricians, neuropediatricians and otorhinolaryngologists) must become aware of the importance of early diagnosis and treatment of OSAS in children[17], which may include the professional category of speech therapists, in order to prevent complications and improve quality of life at this stage of life.

This is because researchers[18] assessed the behaviour of children with OSAS and concluded that neurocognitive, emotional and behavioural difficulties were present in the study sample, highlighting the importance of early diagnosis and intervention. In addition, researchers[19] found that children with excessive daytime sleepiness, one of the characteristics of OSAS, were around ten times more likely to have learning problems.

The impacts of poor sleep

Human sleep is characterised by distinct physiological states that oscillate in 90-minute cycles throughout the night. It is classically divided into REM - paradoxical sleep (Rapid Eye Movement), in which there are rapid eye movements and this phase corresponds to 20% of the total sleep time, and Non REM - slow sleep (Non Rapid Eye Movement - NREM), the phase in which sleep is initiated, with alternation between these two phases[20,21].

It is in NREM sleep that the body recovers from fatigue, synthesises proteins, restores and manufactures cells, antibodies and hormones. REM sleep is where mental fatigue recovers[22].

According to the literature[23], the quantity and quality of sleep affect learning by compromising cognitive functions such as attention and working memory. This is because neural networks related to learning are activated during and after REM and NREM sleep states.

The quality of sleep is due to the harmony between wakefulness and sleep, which favours the proper functioning of various functions, including learning[24]. Therefore, factors that directly interfere with sleep repair can have a detrimental effect on quality of life and learning, as previously stated.

Attention is a cognitive function that allows the focus to be kept on a particular event, thus being called selective attention. When a child is in a classroom and the teacher is explaining a new subject, it is necessary for attention to be selective, i.e. for the focus to be on the explanation given by the teacher and not on the side conversations taking place in the classroom. But if, at a certain moment, two classmates are talking while the teacher is explaining and someone says your name, you also pay attention to what is being said about you - this skill is called divided attention. Thus, one of the factors that can jeopardise this precious cognitive function is non-restorative sleep, which has either been fragmented during the night due to apneas or even for emotional and motivational reasons. As such, this function is a complex one, as it is affected by various factors. Another important aspect to remember is that alterations in attention will consequently affect memory.

Memory, another extremely important cognitive function for learning, is the ability we have to store information in our nervous system that can be useful later on. Its recording depends on the type of stimulus (taste, smell, hearing, visual, tactile or combined sensory stimuli) - because it activates different areas of the brain - and is called sensory memory, which "stores" the information at the moment the stimulus is presented (short-term or working memory) and if this information is useful and is used in the face of the subject's different needs (through control processes. some of which are automatic and others voluntary), it can become useful, some of which are automatic and others voluntary), it can be stored in long-term memory and, when we need the information that has been memorised, it is retrieved for use. The information can become "automatised", so that we use it with a minimum of awareness[25]. From the above, there are several stages necessary so that what we have learnt can be manipulated in the way we want, such as speaking and writing down what we think, for example.

Sleep is the main resource for consolidating newly acquired information in memory. Patterns of neurotransmitters and neurohormones secreted between the different stages of sleep are responsible for consolidating information. While we sleep, proteins are synthesised with the aim of maintaining or expanding the neuronal networks linked to memory and learning[26].

Oliveira[27], in 2012, found that students with healthier sleeping habits tended to be from rural areas, were female and had lower levels of education. He found that as the students got older, their parents gradually decreased their vigilance over the type and time of media use (such as television, telephone, computer games and the internet).

In addition, other external factors, according to the author, influence negative symptoms for a good quality and quantity of sleep, such as brightness in the bedroom; evening walks (like going to the shopping centre, for example); the consumption of caffeinated drinks; an unhealthy diet; behaviour that is not always appropriate (such as pretending to sleep so they can do something without their parents' knowledge). These students admitted to having more difficulties with their memory, attention and concentration, creativity, reasoning, participation in classes and learning, culminating in poorer academic performance.

A study using positron emission tomography showed a global decrease in glucose metabolism covering the entire cortical and subcortical region during sleep deprivation. The subjects who showed the greatest difficulty in solving cognitive tasks were also those who showed the greatest drop in glucose in the prefrontal cortex, thalamus and posterior parietal associative cortex[28].

According to the Brazilian Attention Deficit Disorder Association[29], Attention Deficit/Hyperactivity Disorder (ADHD) occurs in 3 to 5 per cent of children in different provinces of the world where it has been researched. It is believed that several causes may be related to ADHD, but in recent years there has been growing evidence to support the overlap between OSAS and ADHD[30].

ADHD has a high rate of comorbidity with attention disorders and altered respiratory mode, showing its association with low school performance and the presence of oronasal breathing in children and adolescents, regardless of gender, age and type of ADHD diagnosis[31].

Respiratory obstructive factors

The executive functions of attention, concentration and memory, when not performed properly, can impair the brain's ability to function appropriately[32,33], and respiratory obstructive factors should be investigated as possible etiological factors of the problem.

And what can be the causes of mouth breathing?

Mouth breathing can be caused by an upper airway obstruction or by a habit that causes air to pass through the mouth[34]. The main causes of nasopharyngeal obstructive mouth breathing are shown in Table 1 below.

Table 1. Causes of nasal obstruction (adapted from the literature)[35].

Primary		**Secondary**
Physiological	**Non-physiological**	
Constant colds	*Allergic* - seasonal and perennial; *Not allergic;* -/ *Infectious* - acute (for various reasons, including nose *piercing*) or chronic, viral, fungal, parasitic and protozoal; *Non-infectious* *Mechanical* - septal deformity, nasal	'*The post-nasal space* - pharyngeal tonsil hypertrophy and trauma; n *Orepharynx* - hypertrophied palatine tonsils, soft palate with decreased tone e redundant, language base

	septum haematoma, choanal atresia, turbinate hypertrophy, presence of foreign bodies and rhinoliths; Hzperreafiva (idiopathic rhinitis) - imbalance in the autonomic nervous system, hormonal changes, drug induced, chemical irritants and emotional factors; *In Inflammatory* - polyps, sarcoids and granulomas; *Tumour* - presence of tumours (benign, such as angiofibroma and polyp, or malignant) and *D Flow disorders* - atrophic rhinitis and septal perforation.	high (sleep apnoea syndrome); *T Respiratory tract lower* - asthma and chronic obstructive airway disorders; *R Retrognathia and* *R Medicinal rhinitis* - sequelae due to overuse of topical nasal vasoconstrictors.

One of the most common causes of nasal obstruction is tonsillar hyperplasia, which can lead to OSAS, as mentioned above[36]. As a consequence, it results in a series of impairments: poor school performance, cor pulmonale, non-specific behavioural disorders, hyperactivity, daytime sleepiness, distraction and developmental delays, the most serious of which is the weight-statue deficit. The treatment of choice is adenotonsillectomy.

This procedure has shown improvements in respiratory rates during sleep, leading to a positive impact on children's growth, behaviour and cognition[37,38].

In 2006, Weber et al.[39] analysed the incidence of neuropsychological disorders in Brazilian children diagnosed with Obstructive Ventilatory Disorder (OVD) using a *screening* questionnaire and compared the responses before and after surgical treatment (adenotonsillectomy). They concluded that the frequency of neuropsychological disorders in children with OVD was high, more noticeable in younger children through hyperactivity and, in older children, through the other two types (attention/concentration deficit and impulsivity), affecting school performance and socialisation, with neuropsychological improvement after surgery.

Research into mouth breathing and learning disorders

School failure is a phenomenon that affects the whole of Brazilian society, regardless of socio-economic class, and is complex and has multiple causes[40]. Therefore, although this chapter deals with the impact of mouth breathing on learning, other factors must be taken into account when we come across a subject with a learning disorder. The aim of this chapter is for the reader to also consider mouth breathing as a possible cause.

While some researchers have shown that mouth breathing has no impact on learning[41], most have found the opposite, as we'll see below.

The school performance of 33 students with mouth breathing due to obstructive diseases was compared with that of 33 nasal breathing students (control group). The neuropsychological assessment revealed that the mouth breathers' capacity for selective attention, concentration and voluntary attention were lower than the control group. The same occurred in copying and maths tasks[42].

Using a standardised questionnaire on sleep, apnoea and learning and polysomnography in 1494 Hispanic and white schoolchildren, researchers[43] found that there was a higher frequency of sleep disorders, OSAS and learning disorders in Hispanic schoolchildren and that children aged between eight and eleven with learning disorders were more likely to have snoring and excessive daytime sleepiness.

Chedid et al.[44] observed that children with mouth breathing are the ones who are below the expected levels in the literacy process.

Di Francesco et al.[45] found that attention deficit and poor school performance were more prevalent in subjects with tonsillar hypertrophy.

Fensterseifer et al.[46] gathered 48 schoolchildren aged between 8 and 12, with and without learning disabilities, from schools with a low socio-cultural level, and found that the majority of the sample with nasal obstruction (54.2%) also had learning disabilities.

A systematic review study showed that individuals with mouth breathing were more likely to have learning difficulties than those with nasal breathing[47].

Conclusion

In view of the findings, we can conclude that obstructive respiratory factors that lead to mouth breathing can cause learning difficulties, and that this aspect should be taken into account when assessing and dealing with children.

References

1. Palangana IC. Development and learning in Piaget and Vygotsky: the relevance of the social. 6. ed. São Paulo: Summus; 2015.
2. Barriguete C. Affectivity: evolutionary and educational aspects. In: Gonzáles E et al. Specific educational needs. Psychoeducational intervention. Porto Alegre: Artmed; 2007.
3. Silva GA, Giacon LAT. Obstructive sleep apnoea/hypopnoea syndrome (OSAHS). Medicina 2006; 39 (2): 185-94.
4. Silva GA, Sander HH, Eckeli AL, Fernandes RMF, Coelho EB, Nobre F. Basic concepts on obstructive sleep apnoea syndrome. Rev. Bras. Hipertens. 2009; 16(3):150-7.
5. Pereira A. Obstructive sleep apnoea syndrome: pathophysiology, epidemiology, consequences, diagnosis and treatment. Arquivos de Medicina 2007; 21(5/6):159- 73.
6. Zenteno DA, Salinas PF, Vera RU, Brockmann PV, Prado FA. Paediatric Approach to the Study of the Respiratory Trastomes of the Sweat. Rev. chil. pediatr. 2010; 81(5): 445-55.
7. Alexopoulos EI,,Charitos G; Malakasioti G, Varlami V, Gourgoulianis K, Zintzaras E, Kaditis AG. Parental history of adenotonsillectomy is associated with obstructive sleep apnea severity in children with snoring. J Paediatr 2014; 164(6): 1352-7.
8. Kheirandish-Gozal L, Peris E, Gozal D. Vitamin D levels and obstructive sleep apnoea in children. Sleep Med 2014; 15(4): 459-63.
9. Khalyfa A, Serpero LD, Kheirandish-Gozal L, Capdevila OS, Gozal D. TNF-a gene polymorphisms and excessive daytime sleepiness in paediatric obstructive sleep apnea. J Pediatr 2011; 158(1): 77-82.
10. Jennum P, Ibsen R, Kjellberg J. Morbidity and mortality in children with obstructive sleep apnoea: a controlled national study. Thorax 2013; 68(10): 949-54.
11. Ross KR, Storfer-Isser A, Hart MA, Kibler AM, Rueschman M, Rosen CL, Kercsmar CM, Redline S. Sleep-disordered breathing is associated with asthma severity in children. J Paediatr 2012; 160(5): 736-42.

12. Hernández C, Durán-Cantolla J, Lloberes P, González M. Innovations in the epidemiology, natural history, diagnosis and treatment of sleep apnea-hypopnea syndrome. Arch Bronconeumol 2009; 45 Suppl 1: 3-10.

13. Fernandes FMVS, Teles RCVV. Obstructive apnoea syndrome questionnaire in children-18: Portuguese version. Braz. j. otorhinolaryngol. 2013;79(6):720-6.

14. Coté CJ, Posner KL, Domino KB. Death or neurologic injury after tonsillectomy in children with a focus on obstructive sleep apnea: houston, we have a problem! Anesth Analg 2014; 118(6): 1276-83.

15. Fleig AHD. Waiting time for diagnosis and treatment of sleep apnoea syndrome in a Brazilian public hospital. 2013. 79f. Dissertation [Master's in Pneumological Sciences], Universidade Federal do Rio Grande do Sul, Porto Alegre, Rio Grande do Sul, Brazil.

16. Bower C, Buckmiller L. What's new in paediatric obstructive sleep apnea. Curr Opin Otolaryngol Head Neck Surg 2001; 9: 352-8.

17. Balbani APS, Weber SAT, Montovani JC. Update on obstructive sleep apnoea syndrome in childhood. Rev. Bras. Otorrinolaringol. 2005;71(1):74-80.

18. Uema SFH, Vidal MVR, Fujita R, Moreira G, Shirley SNP. Behavioural assessment in children with obstructive sleep disorders. Braz J Otorhinolaryngol. 2006;72(1):120-3.

19. Petry C, Pereira MU, Pitrez P, Jones MH, Stein RT. Prevalence of symptoms of sleep-disordered breathing in Brazilian schoolchildren. J. Pediatr. 2008; 84: 123-9.

20. Rente P, Pimentel T. A pathologia do sono. Lisbon: Lidel; 2004.

21. Marquioli VSF. The influence of sleep on memory and emotion. 2011. Monograph [Specialisation in Neurosciences], Institute of Biological Sciences, Federal University of Minas Gerais, Belo Horizonte.

22. Brunschwig H. Sono. Lisbon: Pergaminho; 2008.

23. Joffily SB, Joffily L, Andraus NM. Sleep state in the learning process. Sciences & Cognition 2014; 19 (3): 531-43.

24. Azevedo DPGD, Azevedo NG. The sound-learning relationship and new information and communication technologies: a challenge in adolescent education. In: Proceedings of the XIII EVIDOSOL and X CILTEC. Universidade Estadual do Norte Fluminense "Darcy Ribeiro" and Universidade Federal Fluminense, Rio de Janeiro, Brazil, June 2016.

25. Boruchovitch E. Learning strategies and school performance: considerations for educational practice. Psicologia Reflexão e Crítica 1999; 12(2): 1-15.
26. Valle LELR, Valle ELR, Reimão R. Sleep and Learning. Rev. Psicopedagogia 2009; 26(80): 286-90.
27. Oliveira OMC. Influence of sleep quality on the health, behaviour and school learning of students in the 2nd and 3rd cycles of basic education. 2012. Master's Degree [Specialisation in Health and Environmental Promotion], University of Minho, Minho, Portugal.
28. Thomas M, Sing H, Belenky G, Holcomb H, Mayberg H, Dannals R et al. Neural basis of alertness and cognitive performance impairments during sleepness. Effects of 24 h of sleep deprivation on waking human regional brain activity. Journal of sleep research 2000; 9: 335-52.
29. Brazilian Attention Deficit Disorder Association. What is ADHD? [Internet site]. Available at http://://www.tdah.org.br/br/sobre-tdah/o-que-eotdah. html>. Consulted on 13/02/2017.
30. Hilario SM, Silva EVCM, Chiloff CLM, Bertoz APM, Micheletti KR, Cuoghi OA, Weber SAT. Neuropsychological disorders and sleep apnoea syndrome in children. Arch Health Invest 2014; 3(3): 65-75.
31. Vera FD, Conde GES, Wajnsztein R, Nemr K. Learning disorder and presence of mouth breathing in individuals diagnosed with attention deficit/hyperactivity disorder (ADHD). Rev. Cefac. 2006;8(4):441-55.
32. Cintra CF, Castro FM, Morato FF, Cintra PP. Orofacial alterations in mouth-breathing patients. Rev Bras Alergia Imunopatol. 2000;23(1): 78-83.
33. Correa BM. Study of the hearing abilities of children with mouth breathing. 2010. Master's Degree [Human Communication Disorders], Federal University of Santa Maria, Santa Maria, Rio Grande do Sul.
34. Bianchini AP, Guedes ZCF, Vieira MM. Study of the relationship between mouth breathing and facial type. Rev Bras Otorrinolaringol 2007; 73(4):500-5.
35. Ianni Filho D, Bertolini MM, Lopes ML. Multidisciplinary contribution to the diagnosis and treatment of nasopharyngeal obstruction and mouth breathing. R Clin Ortodon Dental Press 2006; 4(6): 90-102.

36. Di Francesco RC, Junqueira PA, Frizzarini R, Zerati FE. Weight and height growth after adenotonsillectomy. Rev Bras Otorrinolaringol 2003; 69: 193-6.

37. Montgomery-Downs HE, Crabtree VM, Gozal D. Cognition, sleep and respiration in at-risk children treated for obstructive sleep apnoea. Eur Respir J. 2005; 25(2):336-42.

38. Schechter MS. Technical report: diagnosis and management of childhood obstructive sleep apnea. Paediatrics 2002; 109: e69.

39. Weber SAT, Lima Neto AC, Ternes FJS, Montovani JC. Attention deficit hyperactivity disorder in obstructive sleep apnoea syndrome: is there improvement with surgical treatment? Rev Bras Otorrinolaringol 2006; 72(1): 124-9.

40. Dotti C. School failure in the working classes. In: Grossi EP, Bordin J (Orgs.). Passion for learning. 6ª ed. Petrópolis: Vozes; 1994.

41. Abreu ACB, Morales DA, Ballo MBJF. Mouth breathing influences performance school. Rev Cefac. 2003; 5: 69-73.

42. Godoy MAB. Learning and attention problems in students with upper airway obstruction. 2003. 123f. Dissertation (Master's in Education), State University of Maringá; 2003.

43. Goodwin JL, Babar SI, Kaemingk KL, Rosen GM, Morgan WJ, Sherrill DL, Quan SF. Symptoms related to sleep-disordered breathing in white and Hispanic children: the Tucson Childreifs Assessment of Sleep Apnea Study. Chest J. 2003; 124: 196-203.

44. Chedid KAK, Di Francesco RC, Junqueira PAS. The influence of mouth breathing on the process of learning to read and write in pre-school children. Rev. Psicopedagogia 2004; 21(65): 157-63.

45. Di Francesco RC, Passerotii G, Paulucci B, Miniti A. Mouth breathing in children: different repercussions according to diagnosis. Rev Bras Otorrinolaringol. 2004; 70: 665-70.

46. Fensterseifer GS, Carpes O, Weckx LLM, Martha VF. Mouth breathing in children with learning difficulties. Braz J Otorhinolaryngol. 2013; 79: 620-4.

47. Ribeiro GCA, Santos IDD, Santos ACN, Paranhos LR, César CPHAR. Influence of the breathing pattern on the learning process: a systematic review of literature. Brazilian journal of otorhinolaryngology 2016, 82(4): 466-78.

CHAPTER 4

Breathing and voice

Sonia Coelho

Breathing is a complex process and has been studied in different areas and from various perspectives. It is fundamental for bodily and facial development and for energetic and emotional balance.

From a holistic point of view, as in yoga and Reiki, breathing is referred to as the life force of the universe (Prana, Ki, Chi) and has been shown to benefit the body, mind and spirit when performed in a complete and nasalised way[1]. As such, it dissolves negative energies, reduces anxiety, increases concentration, controls heart flow and rhythm, regulates sleep and the mind.

In psychology, it indicates the rhythms of life, under the influence of our different emotional states. In physiology, it is seen as responsible for gas exchange between the individual and the environment, through inhalation (an active process) and exhalation (a passive process)[(2)].

In Speech and Language Therapy, breathing is common to two specific areas such as Orofacial Motricity and Voice, but has repercussions in others, which is why an assessment of the orofacial structures, the functions of the stomatognathic system and a complete voice assessment are indicated, as well as intervention in both areas.

The primary function of breathing is the exchange of oxygen and carbon dioxide at tissue and lung level through structures that are coordinated with each other, such as the nose, paranasal sinuses, pharynx, larynx, vocal folds, oral cavity (lips, tongue, hard and soft palates, teeth), mandible (upper structures) and lungs, bronchi, bronchioles, abdominal muscles, intercostals, spinal extensors and especially the diaphragm (lower structures)[3,4].

Breathing dynamics involve the modes and types of breathing, the inhale-exhale ratio and the frequency of the cycles, which denote a series of physical and emotional states, and should be calm, regular, deep and harmonious in order to increase the energy and balance of the organism as a whole[5], as is also ratified in Reiki.

The relationship between breathing and the voice is fundamental for its production, more expressive emission through the proper use of body and vocal adjustments, free of tension, in order to avoid possible alterations.

Breathing is life, it's the pulse at birth and the last breath at death.

The topic will then be explored in greater depth in relation to the importance of breathing for vocal production.

The importance of breathing for vocal production

Vocal production occurs through two systems: respiratory and digestive, since there is no specific system for its production. In this sense, breathing is the essential activator from phonation to the process of resonance and projection, since the "raw material" of sound is exhaled air[6].

Breathing is divided into nasal inhalation, which should be almost imperceptible, and exhalation. In singing, exhalation becomes active and is achieved through training, and can be mixed in mode, as in some situations of speech and professional singing[1,7].

In this way, voice involves three processes: initially it is a glottal sound produced by the vibration of the vocal folds, which are located in the larynx. Under the subglottal air pressure coming from the lungs and controlled by the respiratory muscles (aerodynamic component), the vocal folds vibrate (myoelastic component of the vocal fold muscles), producing phonation. Subsequently, this glottal sound is modulated and amplified in the vocal tract or supraglottal tract, which acts as a filter and extends from the vocal folds to the lips (the resonance boxes), at which point it is characterised as voice. The voice then goes through the final process, articulation, in which speech sounds are produced and modified in the oral cavity (by the tongue, teeth, palate and lips)[8].

Breathing can be different depending on our emotional and physical state and the way we use it. In colloquial spoken voice, inhalation is rapid and can be oral, with passive exhalation and little chest expansion, making it more spontaneous and natural. The focus is on articulation, directed towards transmitting the content, which is the goal. In professional spoken voice, exhalation is related to the content, speed and articulation of the words and depends on the length of the sentences, the individual's emotion and intention, making breathing training appropriate. The content is the focus and must be expressed in such a way as to reach the other person. In the singing voice, training is crucial because exhalation is active, with great chest expansion and conditioned by melodic phrases, rhythm, pauses and other musical and interpretative aspects. Here, form is the focus, and articulatory precision can be reduced[9].

Control of breathing and vocal techniques is essential for the professional singing voice. The differences are accentuated in the popular or classical singing voice, which has very unique characteristics and demands[10].

The method of muscle and joint chains (Godelieve Denys-Struyf - G.D.S.) studied by Steuer and Ferreira[11] showed that the absence of vocal alterations is the result of the relationship between body expression, breathing, emotion and the subject's own voice. In this way, the authors considered vocal production to be dependent on the psyche and the harmony between breathing, tension and muscular rhythm. Voice, body and breathing become inseparable and tensions lead to a rigid system that must be avoided in order not to cause vocal disorders. Pneumophono-articulatory coordination must include rhythm, appropriate body positions and expressions, as well as breathing flexibility.

Researchers[12] have shown that the coordination of the laryngeal muscles (extrinsic and intrinsic) allows for efficient vocal production, since the extrinsic muscles influence the intrinsic muscles, playing an important role in the respiratory, digestive, phonatory and articulatory systems and, consequently, altering the shape and tension of the vocal folds, frequency, intensity, subglottal pressure, resonance and vocal register, which are fundamental for inspiration, speech and singing.

Breathing work is more widespread in singing, due to its demands and specificities, especially with regard to respiratory support (used in singing) which allows for correct adjustments of head and body postures; relief of body and laryngeal tensions; respiratory control through airflow balance and consequent pneumophonoarticulatory coordination; mastery, power and stability in vocal emission; greater capacity for sustaining phrases; increased proprioception;

improved projection; aesthetic quality of the voice; resonance flexibility and expressiveness, providing longevity and vocal health[7]. Although there are inconsistencies in terms of nomenclature, strategies and the most appropriate types of breathing support (costal, diaphragmatic, abdominal, together or in parts), the training more specifically involves the abdominal and intercostal muscles.

Cielo et al.[13] also reported that the nasal and mixed modes were the most used by the subjects in their study, but they considered the latter to be inappropriate for voice professionals, due to their vocal needs. The authors recognised that this is an aspect that requires speech therapy intervention, as it involves guidance on voice care and training in the most appropriate type of breathing (costo-diaphragmatic-abdominal) to prevent vocal disorders. They also commented on the difficulty of obtaining studies on breathing patterns for these professionals.

The assessment and preparation of voice professionals should include training in pneumophono-articulatory coordination, as this can reduce the occurrence of dysphonia caused by pneumophono-articulatory incoordination[14].

As for breathing types, they can be categorised as: clavicular or upper (with less air intake, shallow inspiration, noisy, cervical and laryngeal tensions), middle/mixed or thoracic, (used in colloquial speech and at rest, without great effort and energy expenditure), lower or abdominal (with little energy) and complete/diaphragmatic-abdominal or costo-diaphragmatic-abdominal (with harmonic expansion of the entire rib cage, requiring training due to the large air intake, in order to avoid tensions). The most suitable type is the costo-diaphragmatic-abdominal, which allows for adequate lung ventilation, intake and phonation, without strain and tension for the speaking and singing voice[1].

Proper breathing should preferably be done through the nasal passage, where the air is filtered, humidified and heated, with lip sealing[4].

Remember that alternating air permeability of the nostrils is a physiological process considered normal.

The so-called pneumophonoarticulatory coordination (PAPC) involves the interaction between breathing (air pressure), phonation (vibration of the vocal folds), articulation and resonance (modified by the vocal tract), allowing proper use of the voice, reducing tension and providing a more appropriate body posture.

After reviewing the main concepts and fundamental processes necessary for healthy vocal production, the impacts of mouth breathing on the voice will be explained.

The impact of mouth breathing on the voice

When breathing occurs in the oral or mixed form, a series of negative repercussions are noted, as already mentioned in previous chapters.

In this chapter, the focus is on the impact of mouth breathing on vocal production.

Among the structural alterations that can have a negative impact on development are craniofacial alterations (long and narrow face due to vertical growth, narrow nostrils, ogival and atretic palate, underdeveloped maxilla, occlusal alterations), postural alterations (alterations to the body axis, lip seal, the usual position of the tongue - on the floor of the mouth and on the lips, with the lower tongue inverted and the upper tongue short and elevated), those related to tone (with a decrease in the muscles of the lips and tongue) and hydration (dry lips and mucous membranes)[15], all of which, in one way or another, can interfere with voice production, as will be seen below.

One of the difficulties cited in the literature for mouth-breathing patients in relation to their voice concerns vocal intensity, especially in communicative activities that require greater vocal intensity, and there have been reports of impairment in this type of task[16,17].

As vocal alterations usually occur due to hypertrophy of the palatine tonsils, these can reduce the movement of the soft palate and modify the morphology, posture and tone of the tongue as well, leading, among other things, to pneumophonoarticulatory incoordination[4,16], in other words, interfering with the perceptual quality of the voice and also increasing complaints such as tiredness when speaking.

Another impact is on resonance, generating a voice with hyper- or hyponasal sonority or a hoarse vocal quality. There are still few publications discussing the relationship between mouth breathing and dysphonia[18,19].

The following vocal alterations have also been found in mouth breathers: velar coupling with denasal adjustment, articulation that tends towards labiodentalisation, vocal quality that can vary from hoarse, breathy to harsh, consequently reducing vocal stability[16] and a lower fundamental frequency[19].

In addition to the above, it should be emphasised that the voice emitted with effort is related to breathing, posture, laryngeal movements, resonance boxes and articulation, all of which produce tension and possible dysphonia.

Speech therapy and interdisciplinary intervention

Since breathing is the "fuel" of vocal production, specialist intervention is indicated, as most people don't use it properly. Therefore, understanding the anatomy and physiology of breathing; the causes, signs and symptoms of possible respiratory alterations; working together with ENT, dentistry, orthodontics, nutrition, physiotherapy, psychology and speech therapy are fundamental for correct diagnoses and interventions. In some cases, surgery and the use of medication are necessary, but the habit of mouth breathing can remain, in which case reassessment and therapy are essential.

Intervention begins with a careful anamnesis involving the complaint, family and professional history, general and specific health history (aspects of the patient's Orofacial Motricity, Language, Hearing and Voice), previous therapies, assessment of the structures of the nasal and oral cavity (morphology, colour, symmetry, tone, positions, size, volume, thickness and praxis), stomatognathic functions with audiovisual recordings and photographs and referrals to related professionals for other assessments and specific tests such as: rhinopharyngeal radiography, lateral teleradiography and nasofibroscopy among others, thus obtaining the correct assessment and prognosis, due to the multifactorial cause of mouth breathing.

Despite the above, the literature[20] has reported that there are few studies that integrate mouth breathing and professionals from other areas of health and also research that relates body posture to the stomatognathic system in mouth breathers.

In vocal assessment specifically, in addition to the above, it is important to know vocal behaviour and use, eating habits, deleterious and vicious habits, general illnesses, previous alterations, followed by perceptual-auditory and acoustic analysis, for vocal diagnosis.

Due to the subjectivity and diversity of cases, in general the perceptual-auditory evaluation of the voice can involve the following aspects: vocal quality, pitch, loudness, respiratory dynamics (type: upper or thoracic, middle or costo-diaphragmatic and lower: abdominal and mode: nasal, oral and mixed), pneumophonarticulatory coordination, phonatory measures, body posture, articulation, resonance, vocal attack and resistance, vocal extension and projection, speed and rhythm of speech, emphases, inflections and pauses. In acoustic analysis, the following aspects can be checked: fundamental frequency, average intensity, formants, jitter, shimmer, noise measurements, among others, in both spontaneous and automatic speech and reading tasks[2].

Before starting the actual treatment, the etiological factor causing the mouth breathing must be resolved and, in the case of allergic rhinitis, the patient and family (in the case of children) must be made aware of the possibility of recurrences when there is exposure to allergenic factors.

Explaining to the patient how the voice is produced and the proper use of the stomatognathic structures and functions that are part of the process, since the voice is a product of the nervous, respiratory and digestive systems, is fundamental, as well as focusing on vocal behaviour, in which issues related to organic, psychological, environmental, social and cultural components characterise the subject's vocal dynamics and identity.

Guidance and care with the use of the voice, hydration, vocal warming up and cooling down are all part of the therapy, contextualised with the patient's use of it, with techniques and methods applied to their diagnosis.

As for breathing, we must make sure that the air is properly permeabilised, preferably nasally (mode), by cleaning the nose properly and using a Glatzel mirror at the beginning and end of the session. Inhalation with warm water or saline solution can be recommended, as well as stimulating the sense of smell and taste, which are diminished in mouth breathers, seeking to improve the posture and tone of the structures (jaw, tongue and lips) through massage and working on the proprioception of the facial muscles and adjusting the functions (swallowing, chewing, speaking and restoring respiratory function), according to the literature[4].

It is worth pointing out that postural and physical conditioning, which are generally altered in these cases, should be worked on and physiotherapists should be consulted, as they interfere with vocal production, such as the position of the head, shoulders, scapulae and abdomen, bearing in mind the influence of the extrinsic muscles of the larynx and the muscles that are part of the breathing process.

Guimarães[21] stated that vocal intervention can involve general and specific relaxation techniques, postural control versus breathing, auditory discrimination and vocal control in different vocal behaviours.

In addition, working with costo-diaphragmatic-abdominal breathing can be achieved through conditioning and training with fricatives and vowels, allowing for more adequate breathing, stipulating times, with support for the spoken and sung voice, for voice and communication professionals, being a practice that comes from singing and is still used in speech therapy.

According to Behlau et al.[2], work in the field of voice has started to carry out fewer extensive tests in relation to breathing (except in some cases), with more emphasis on assessing pneumophonoarticulatory coordination, glottal sonorisation and speech articulation. For the authors, the literature does not confirm that dysphonia is the result of an inadequate or incorrect breathing pattern. However, in clinical practice we have seen the value of working with both the type and mode of breathing in dysphonia and the importance of working on vocal aspects in mouth breathers.

Proper breathing should be worked on throughout the therapeutic process: in the warm-up and vocal cool-down, in the techniques and methods used in the sessions. It should also be remembered that most of the techniques used in the area of voice originated in singing and many of them focus on posture, relaxation, breathing, resonance, voice projection and articulation, seeking an effortless vocal emission, especially for voice professionals.

Final considerations

It was found that there is a close relationship between the anatomical structures and functions that make up breathing and vocal production, which also influences behaviour and vocal quality. Knowing the mechanisms of breathing and voice is therefore essential, as once they are maladjusted they can lead to vocal disorders.

Respiratory alterations have multifactorial etiologies and diverse consequences that characterise the need for interdisciplinary intervention, the treatment of which must be individualised and based on correct diagnosis in order to prevent major sequelae, with the aim of rebalancing the entire system and, to this end, must involve different professionals.

Breathing is therefore correlated with most vocal parameters, body posture and emotional states. The differences between oral breathing for speaking and singing were evident, the latter being dependent on training and time. Furthermore, mastery of breathing is essential for voice and communication professionals.

Nasal breathing leads to adequate growth and development of stomatognathic structures and functions, as well as allowing for more efficient vocal production and should be encouraged. The oral or mixed breathing mode, on the other hand, in addition to insufficient ventilation, is more prone to triggering maladjustments in voice parameters, causing possible dysphonia.

Although breathing is the basis of vocal production, few studies have related it to the voice, whether used for colloquial, professional or sung speech. There was also disagreement among professionals as to the most appropriate type of breathing support, although the costo-diaphragmatic-abdominal type was recommended due to the guaranteed air supply for vocal production and the fact that the studies were more focused on voice professionals.

We conclude that there is a relationship between mouth breathing and dysphonia, and that it is of the utmost importance for the speech therapist to assess and work on Orofacial Motricity and Voice, due to the intimacy of their structures and functions. It is also essential to invest in and publicise therapeutic strategies for breathing (upper airway) and support (lower airway) that are best suited to the needs of each patient. It was noted that there is a need for more studies on this subject and for interdisciplinary intervention, as it has always been more studied by singing teachers. It can be said that nasal breathing is essential for human communication and for an adequate quality of life, and should be investigated in the event of complaints or observation of phonoaudiological alterations.

References

1. Oliveira MC. Various breathing techniques for singing. [monograph] Salvador: CEFAC; 2000.

2. Behlau M, Madazio G, Feijó D, Pontes, P. Voice Assessment. In: Behlau M. (Org.) Voice. The specialist's book, v. 1. Rio de Janeiro: Revinter; 2001. p. 85-180.

3. Souchard PE. Breathing. São Paulo: Summus; 1989.

4. Marchesan IQ. Assessment and therapy of breathing problems. In: Marchesan IQ (Org.). Fundamentos de fonoaudiologia: aspectos clínicos da motricidade oral. 2. ed. Rio de Janeiro: Guanabara Koogan; 2005. p. 29-43.

5. Behlau MS, Pontes PAL. Voice assessment. In: Behlau MS, Pontes PAL. Assessment and treatment of dysphonia. São Paulo: Lovise; 1995. p. 106-17.

6. Pinho SMR. Voice assessment and treatment. In: Pinho SMR. Fundamentals of Speech Therapy: treating voice disorders. Rio de Janeiro: Guanabara Koogan; 1998. p. 3-37.

7. Gava Júnior W, Ferreira LP, Andrada e Silva MA. Respiratory support in the singing voice: perspectives of singing teachers and speech therapists. Rev CEFAC 2010; 12(4): 551-62.

8. Pinho SMR, Tsuji DH, Bohadana AC. Laryngeal physiology. In: Pinho, SMR, Tsuji DH, Bohadana AC. Fundamentals of laryngology and voice. Rio de Janeiro: Revinter; 2006. p. 1-20.

9. Behlau M, Feijó D, Madazio G, Rheder MI, Azevedo R, Ferreira AE. Professional voice: General aspects of speech therapy. In: Behlau M. (Org.) Voice. The specialist's book, v. 2. Rio de Janeiro: Revinter; 2005. p. 287-407.

10. Oliveira SCC de. Roberto Carlos' voice: perceptual-auditory evaluation, acoustic analysis and the public's opinion. [dissertation] São Paulo: PUCSP; 2007.

11. Steuer F, Ferreira LP. Clinical vocal expression: dysphonia and fixity. Distúrb Comum 2008; 20(3): 307-17.

12. Peter GS, Pinho SMR, Assencio-Ferreira, VJ. Extrinsic muscles of the larynx and their participation in vocal production. Rev CEFAC 2001; 3: 165-73.

13. Cielo CA, Hoffman CF, Scherer T, Christmann MK. Breathing type and mode of future voice professionals. Rev Saúde 2013; 39(1): 121-30.

14. Cielo CA, Christmann MK, Scherer TM, Hoffman CF. Airflow adapted to phonic coefficients of future voice professionals. Rev CEFAC 2014; 16(2): 54653.

15. Planas P. Reabilitação neuroclusal. 2. ed. Rio de Janeiro: Medsi; 1998.

16. Denunci, FV. Mouth breathing and vocal quality in childhood: a comparative study. [dissertation] São Paulo: Pontifical Catholic University of São Paulo; 2003.

17. Campanha SMA, Fontes MJF, Santos JLF. Dyspnoea in individuals with asthma, allergic rhinitis and mouth breathing. Rev CEFAC 2012; 14(2): 268-73.

18. Tavares JG, Silva ÉHAA. Theoretical considerations on the relationship between mouth breathing and dysphonia. Rev Soc Bras Fonoaudiol 2008; 13(4): 405-10.

19. Viegas D, Viegas F, Atherino CCT, Baeck HE. Voice spectral parameters in mouth breathing children. Rev CEFAC 2010; 12(5): 820-30.

20. Machado PG, Mezzomo CL, Badaró AFV. Body posture and stomatognathic functions in mouth-breathing children: a literature review. Rev CEFAC 2012; (14): 553-65.

21. Guimarães I. Voice problems in teachers: prevalence, causes, effects and forms of prevention. Rev Portuguesa de Saúde Pública 2004; 22(2): 33-41.

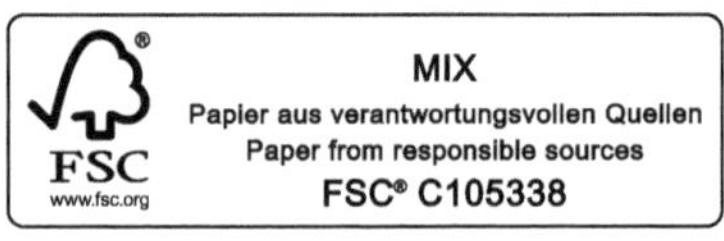

Printed by Books on Demand GmbH, Norderstedt / Germany